live

**artful messages
of hope, happiness
& healing**

**BY
ERIC SMITH
& FRIENDS**

now

**HOW
BOOKS**

Cincinnati, Ohio
www.howdesign.com

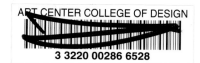

For more excellent books and resources for designers, visit www.howdesign.com.

15 14 13 12 11   5 4 3 2 1

Distributed in Canada by Fraser Direct, 100 Armstrong Avenue, Georgetown, Ontario, Canada L7G 5S4, Tel: (905) 877-4411. Distributed in the U.K and Europe by F+W Media International, Brunel House, Newton Abbot, Devon, TQ12 4PU, England, Tel: (+44) 1626-323200, Fax: (+44) 1626-323319, E-mail: postmaster@davidandcharles.co.uk. Distributed in Australia by Capricorn Link, P.O. Box 704, Windsor, NSW 2756 Australia, Tel: (02) 4577-3555.

Library of Congress Cataloging-in-Publication Data

Smith, Eric.
 Live now / Eric Smith. -- 1st ed.
    p. cm.
 Includes index.
 ISBN 978-1-4403-0841-3 (pbk. : alk. paper)
 1. Conduct of life--Quotations, maxims, etc. I. Title.
 BJ1581.2.S565 2011
 170'.44--dc22
                                 2010045262

Edited by Megan Patrick
Cover designed by Eric Smith
Interior designed by Grace Ring
Production coordinated by Greg Nock

ABOUT THE AUTHOR

Eric Smith was born and raised in a small town in the Pacific Northwest, you've probably never heard of it. Thankfully, he didn't have to look far for inspiration. When you're surrounded by trees bigger than your house, and every direction you turn looks like a rocky mountain postcard, you're in Washington. Other early inspirations as an 80's kid include: Nickelodeon, BMX culture and his Dad's record collection. Through the love and encouragement of his Mom, Smith's hands were never far from a sketchpad and pencil. High five, Mom!

Spring 2008 brought more than a change of season. Along with the rain came a flood when Smith was diagnosed with cancer. Life would never be the same, but that was for the better. He began to discover what cancer could gift to him—the ability to absorb each moment as if it were his whole life. Smith began creating as a method of healing; optimism and hand drawn typography made for the perfect antidote. What was once a seed became a fruit, and people from all over the globe started to hear about Live Now and wanted to join in on the fun. Today, there is a strong community of more than 100 friends pursuing the present and spreading happiness.

Alongside Live Now, Eric Smith runs IDRAWALLDAY, a freelance graphic design, illustration, and art direction practice. To learn more about the author visit www.idrawallday.com.

**Dedicated to the source
of true happiness and love.**

introduction

Some time ago, I was diagnosed with cancer. Instantly perspective changed within me. The fearful, human part of my being wanted to resist this disease, label it as bad and be at the mercy of this situation. But the essence of my spirit knew that this situation could not be isolated from the hidden harmony I seek to follow each day. Having my physical life threatened provoked within me a strong separation between my spiritual and physical being. Although my physical body was being attacked, my spiritual essence was untouchable.

My experience with cancer was this: Live Now! Cancer changed the way I ate, slept, and most important, the way I live. Before cancer I was like most folks, just cruising along. It was during my treatment when I started to discover what cancer could gift to me—the ability to absorb every moment as if each one were my whole life. The Live Now Project was born!

We are a growing collection of friends powerfully pursuing the notion of living now. We're spreading our message through artwork, literature, relationships, exhibitions and more. This movement cannot be confined, is spilling out, and making history. The Live Now book is a selection of artwork from myself and many other talented friends from around the world. We hope you enjoy it.

Find out more at **www.welivenow.org.**

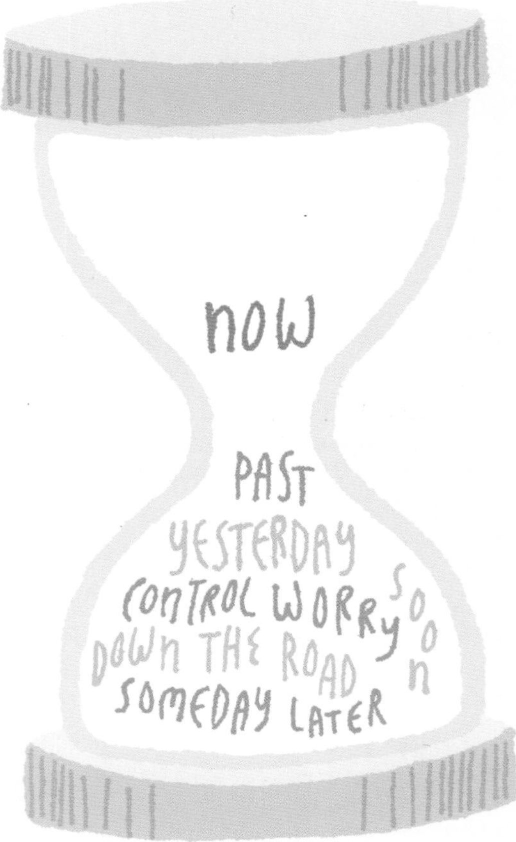
NOW
PAST
YESTERDAY
CONTROL WORRY
SOON
DOWN THE ROAD
SOMEDAY LATER

live now
www.welivenow.org

/

ERIC SMITH
www.idrawallday.com

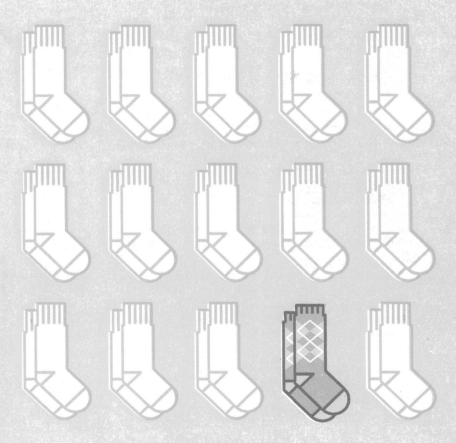

BREAK YOUR ROUTINE

live now

MIKEY BURTON
www.mikeyburton.com

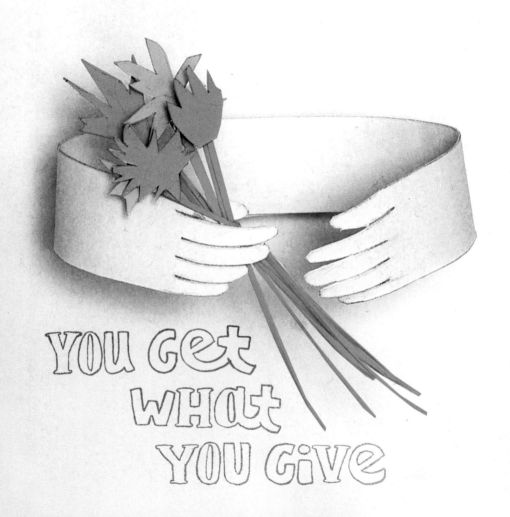

live now
www.welivenow.org

/

SLIDE SIDEWAYS
www.slide-sideways.com

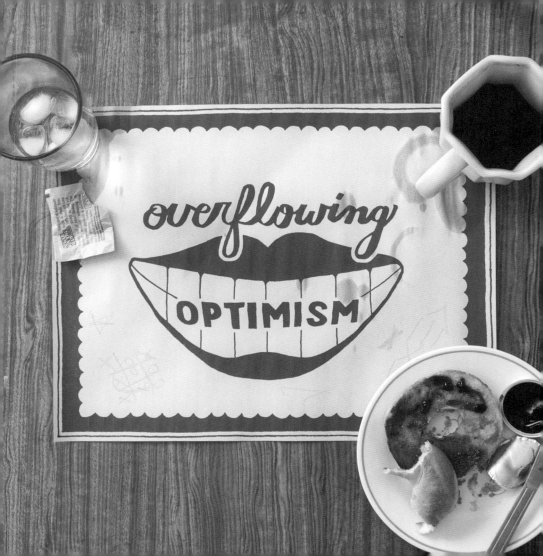

live now
www.welivenow.org

/

CHAD KOURI
www.longliveanalog.com, www.thepostfamily.com
Photo by Ben Speckmann

HARMONY

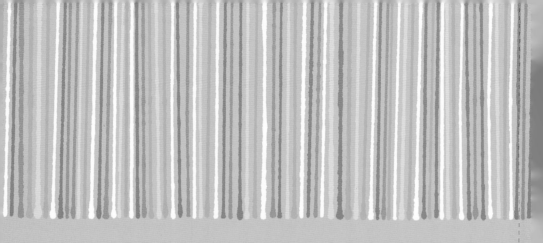

live now
www.welivenow.org

/

ERIC SMITH
www.idrawallday.com

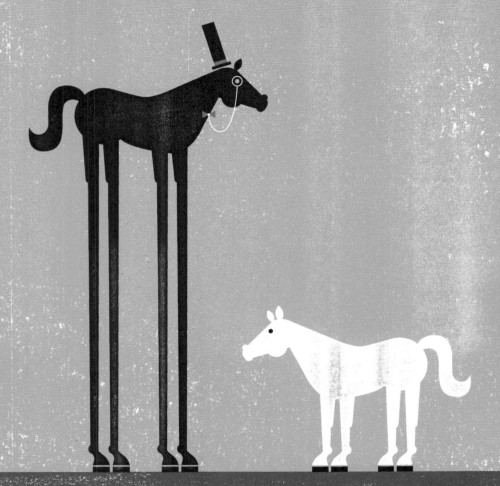

LIVE HUMBLY

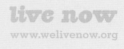

www.welivenow.org

/

MIKEY BURTON
www.mikeyburton.com

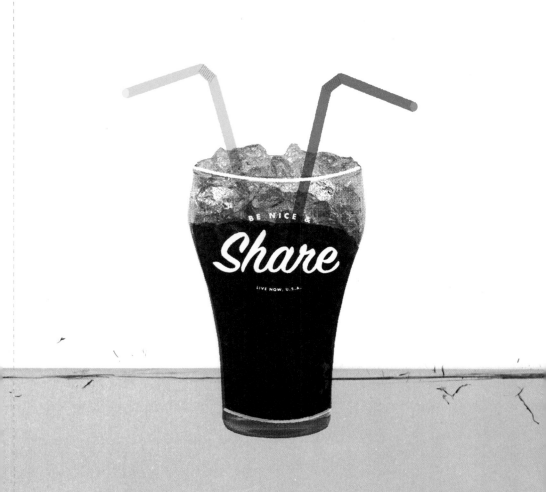

live now

www.welivenow.org

/

AARON BOUVIER

www.aaronbouvier.com

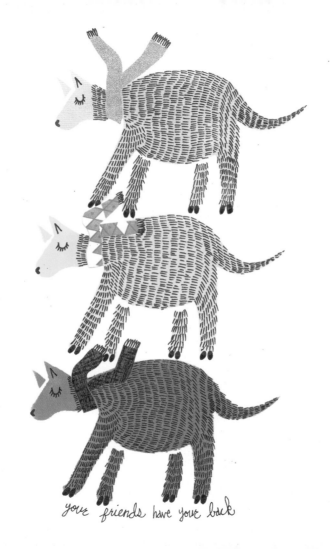

your friends have your back

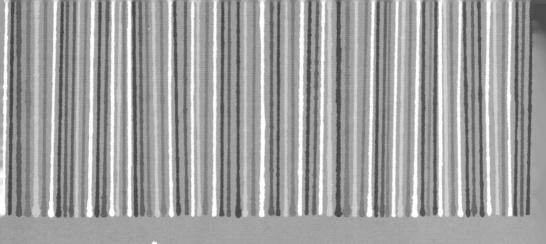

live now
www.welivenow.org

TY WILLIAMS
www.typaints.com

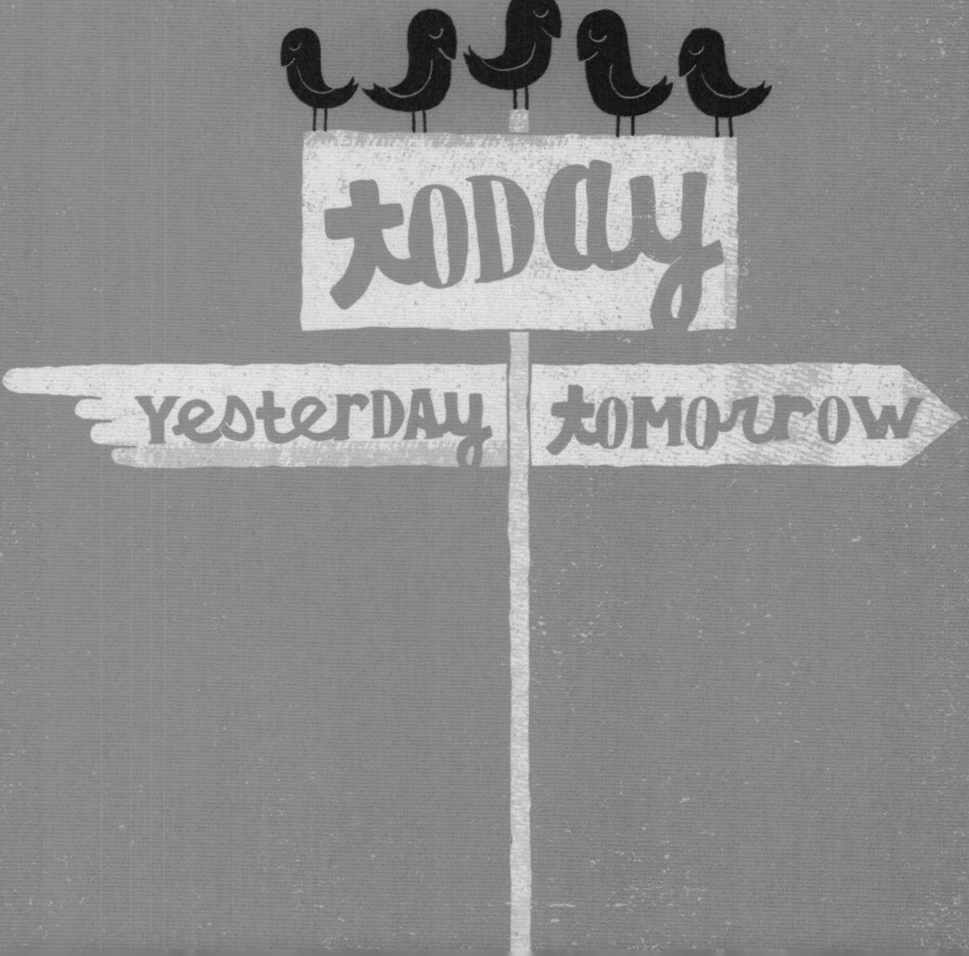
today
yesterday
tomorrow

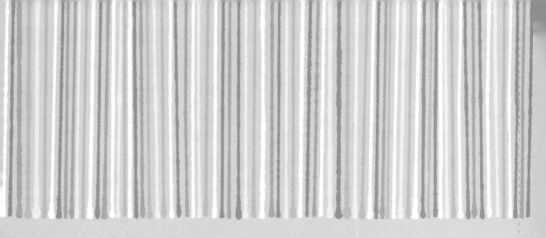

live now
www.welivenow.org

/

SLIDE SIDEWAYS
www.slide-sideways.com

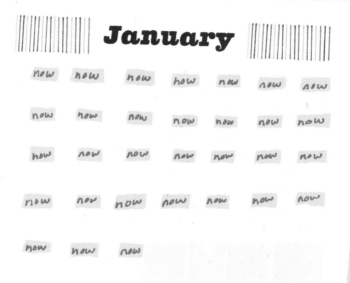

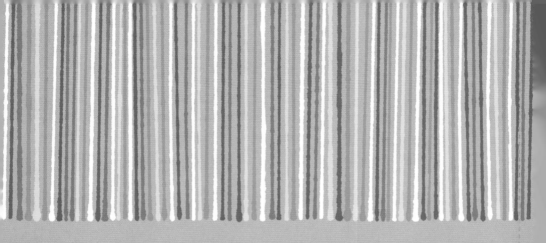

live now
www.welivenow.org

ERIC SMITH
www.idrawallday.com

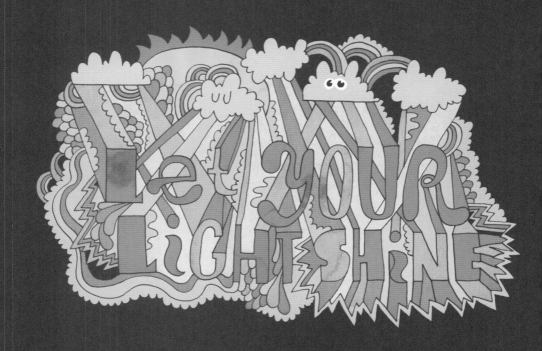

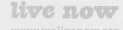
www.welivenow.org

WILL BRYANT
www.willbryant.com

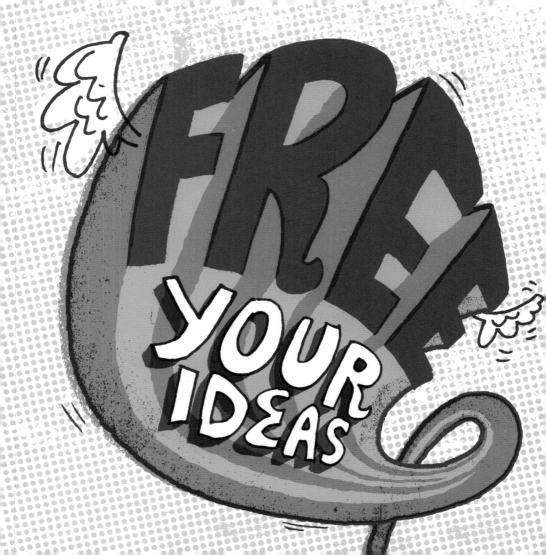

live now
www.welivenow.org

ANDY SMITH
www.asmithillustration.com

HIGHER FIVES

LIVE
NOW

live now
www.welivenow.org

/

ED NACIONAL
ednacional.com

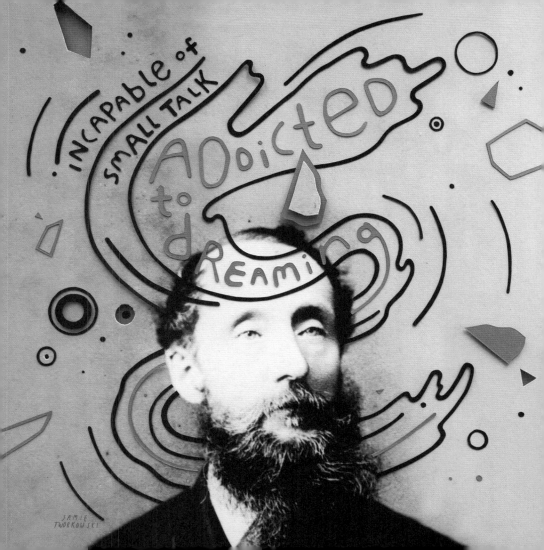

INCAPABLE of SMALL TALK

ADDICTED to dREAMing

JAMIE TWORKOWSKI

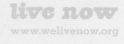

OWEN GILDERSLEEVE

www.owengildersleeve.com

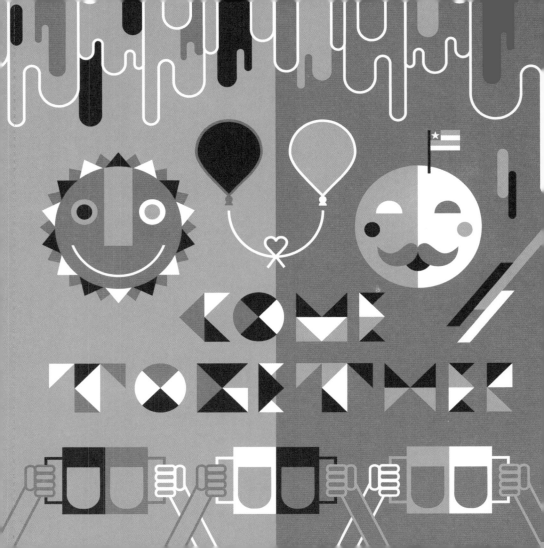

live now
www.welivenow.org

/

J. BYRNES
www.adapt-studio.com

KEEP ON EXPLORING

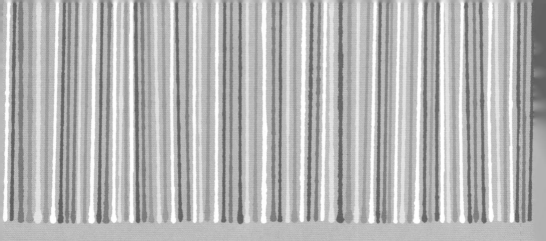

live now
www.welivenow.org

/

RICHARD PEREZ
www.skinnyships.com

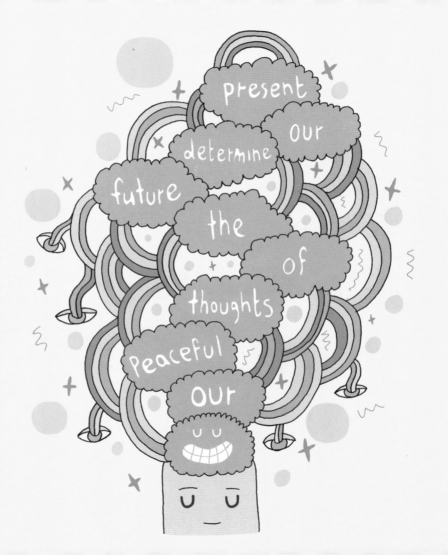

live now
www.welivenow.org

/

MATTHEW DENT
www.matthewdent.co.uk

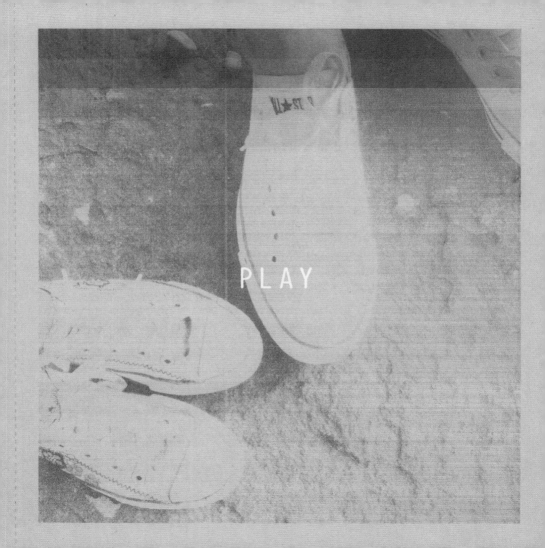

live now
www.welivenow.org

/ **ERIC SMITH**
www.idrawallday.com

LIVE WITH A FRESH HEART

live now

BEN ASLETT

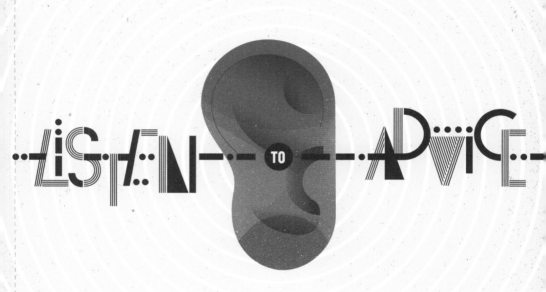

LISTEN TO ADVICE

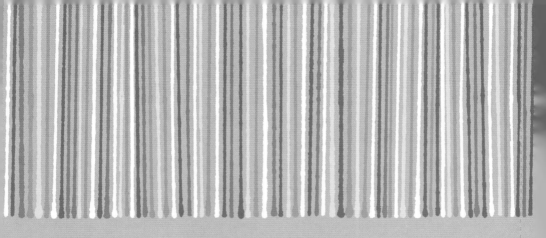

live now
www.welivenow.org

/

RICHARD PEREZ
www.skinnyships.com

SEEK GOOD

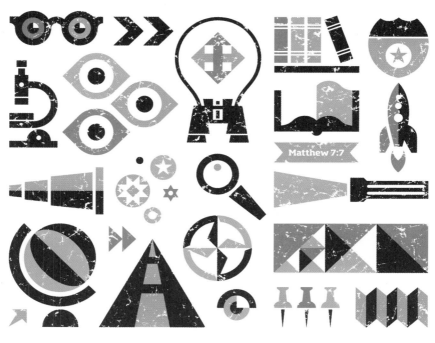

Matthew 7:7

live now
www.welivenow.org

TY WILKINS
tywilkins.com

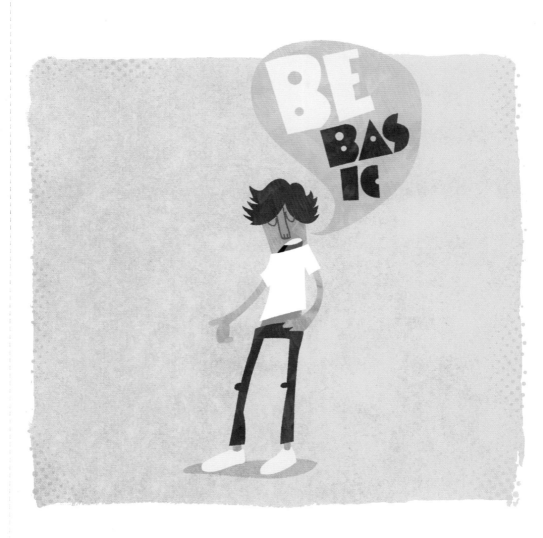

live now
www.welivenow.org

BRIAN GOSSETT
www.theartofdoingsomething.com

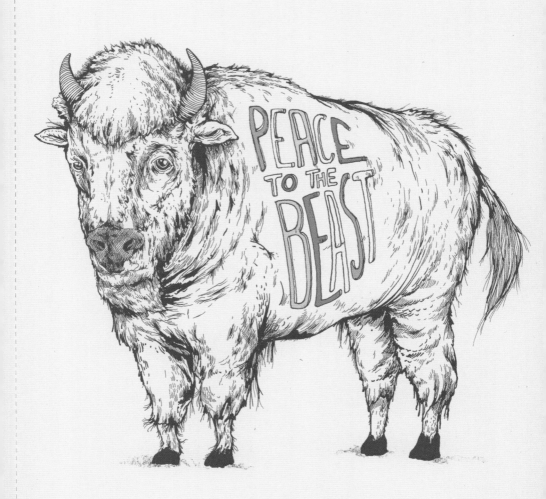

live now
www.welivenow.org

/

PAT PERRY
www.patperry.net

Calm & Collected

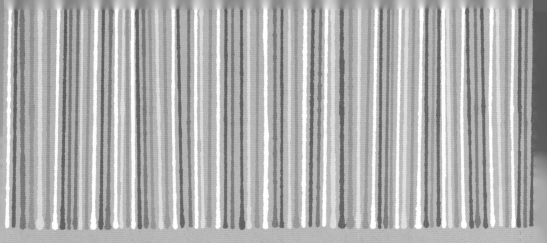

live now
www.welivenow.org

DAN CASSARO
www.YoungJerks.com

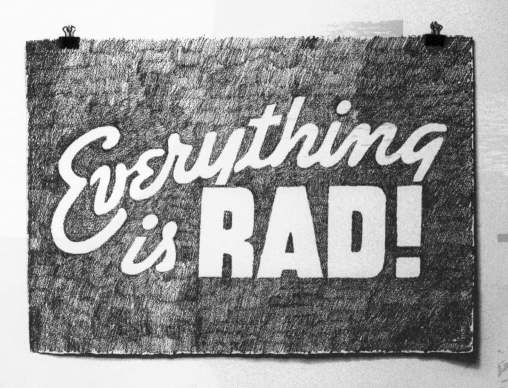

live now
www.welivenow.org

NICK ZEGEL
www.nickzegel.com, www.zeegisbreathing.com

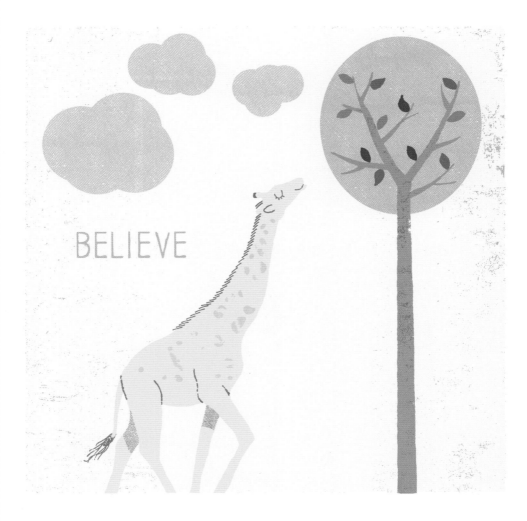

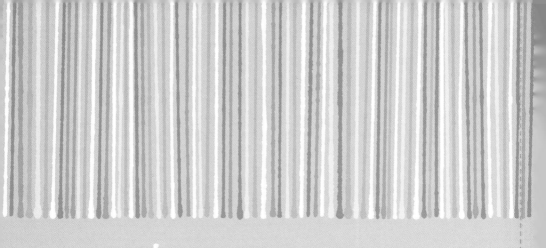

live now
www.welivenow.org

/

SEAN SUTHERLAND
www.madebysean.com

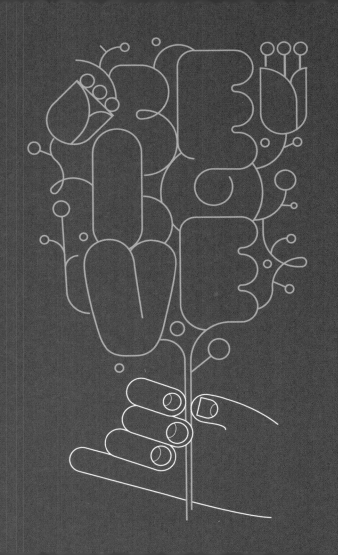

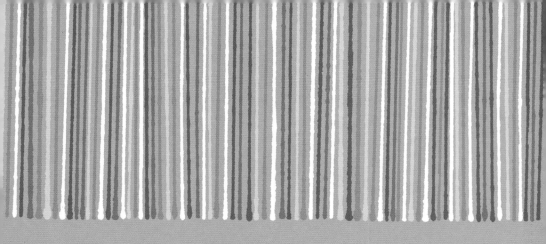

live now
www.welivenow.org

/

JONATHAN CALUGI
www.happyloverstown.eu

S

BUE

EMV!

SME

TER

R

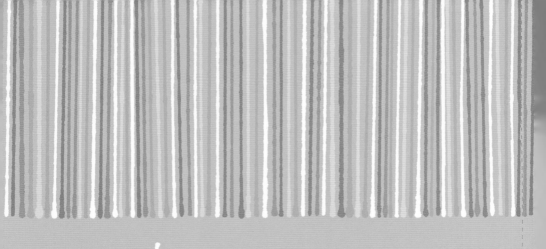

live now
www.welivenow.org

J. ZACHARY KEENAN
www.j-zachary.com

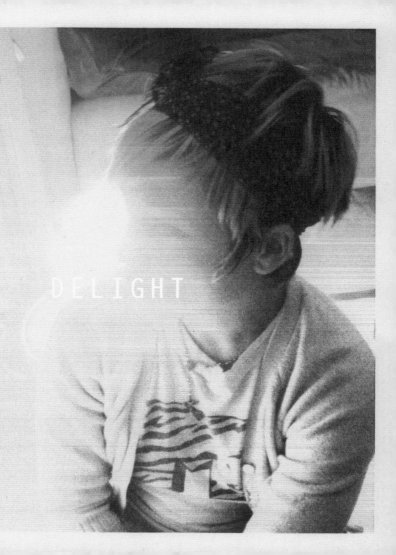

DELIGHT

live now

ERIC SMITH

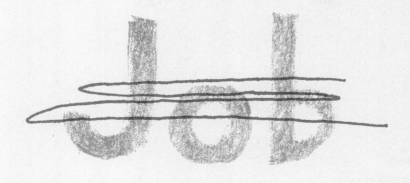

CALLING

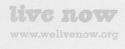

ERIC SMITH

www.idrawallday.com

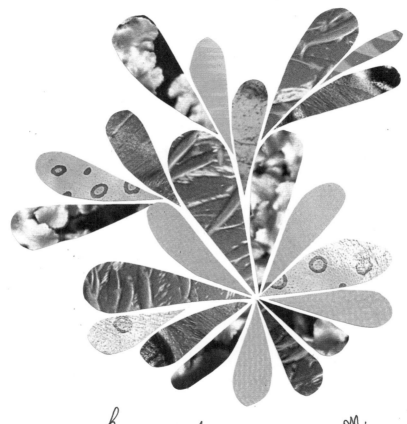

keep calm and carry on

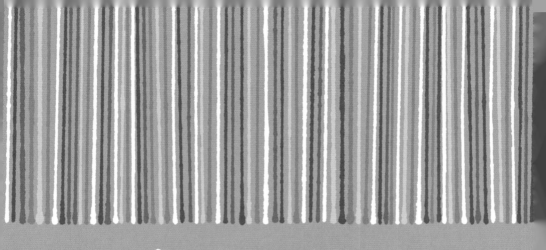

live now
www.welivenow.org

/

TY WILLIAMS
www.typaints.com

LESS ADJECTIVES MORE VERBS

live now
www.welivenow.org

ERIC SMITH
www.idrawallday.com

EASY
GOING

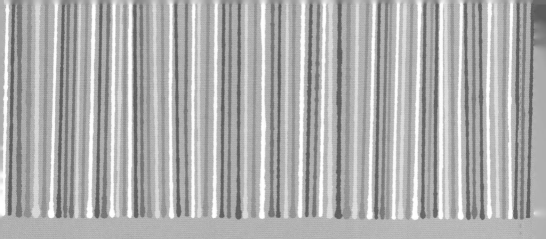

live now
www.welivenow.org

/

ERIC SMITH
www.idrawallday.com

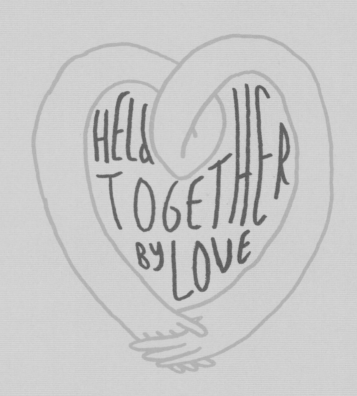

live now
www.welivenow.org

ERIC SMITH
www.idrawallday.com

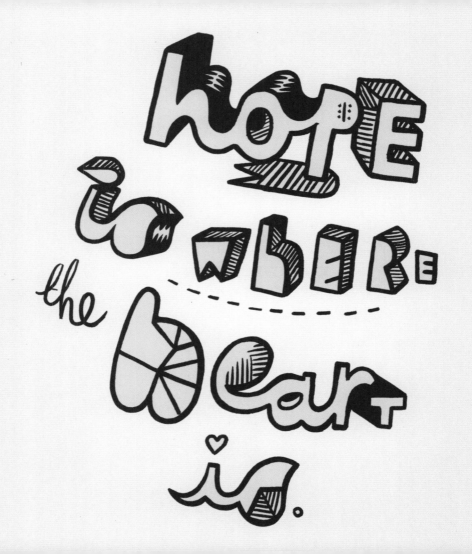

live now

/

NICK DEAKIN
www.nickdeakin.com

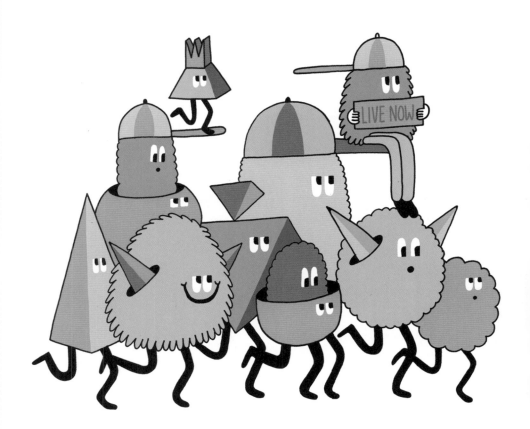

live now / **MATTHEW DENT**
www.welivenow.org www.matthewdent.co.uk

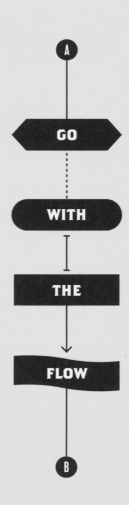

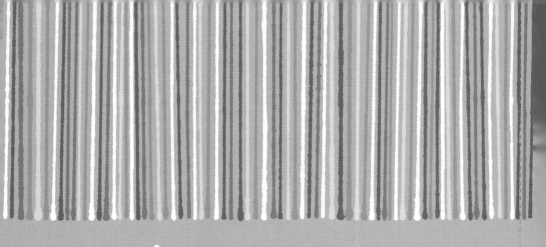

live now / **LOZ IVES**

www.welivenow.org www.becausestudio.co.uk

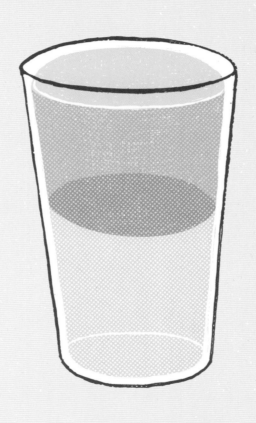

live now
www.welivenow.org

/

JESSE HORA
www.jessehora.com

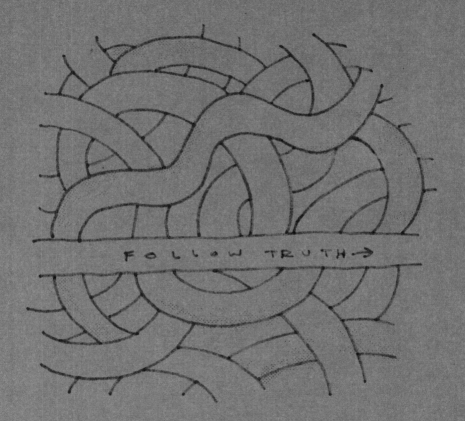

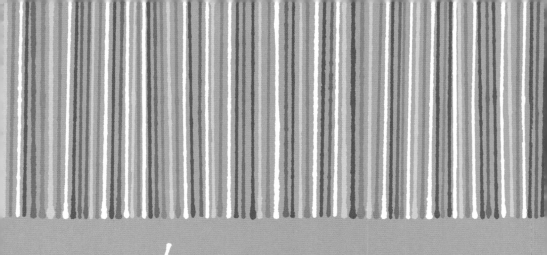

live now / **ERIC SMITH**

www.welivenow.org / www.idrawallday.com

YOU'RE GOING PLACES

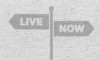

live now
www.welivenow.org

/

ED NACIONAL
ednacional.com

THE SURE THING BOAT NEVER GETS FAR FROM SHORE

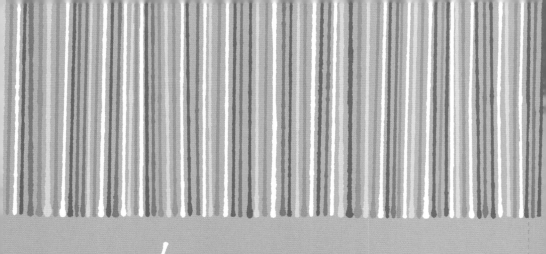

live now
www.welivenow.org

/

JEFFREY BOWMAN
www.mrbowlegs.co.uk

Stay STRONG

live now
www.welivenow.org

/

ADAM R GARCIA
www.thepressure.org

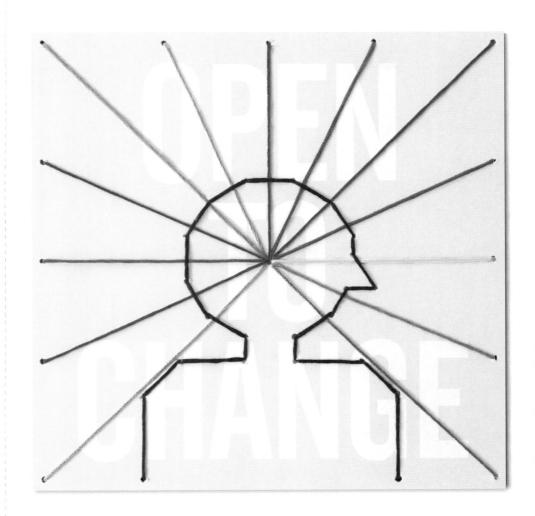

STEPHEN KELLEHER

www.frankenstyles.com

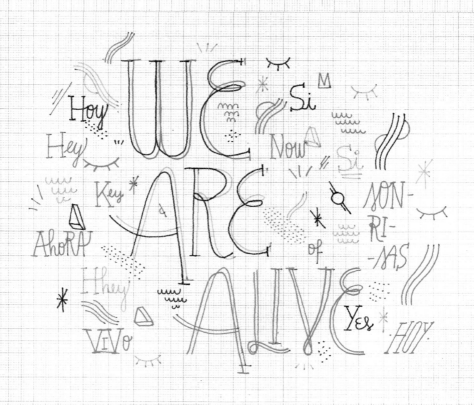

live now

BOSQUE STUDIO

happy
people
humm...

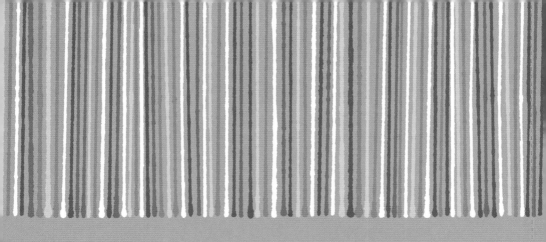

live now
www.welivenow.org

/

ERIC SMITH
www.idrawallday.com

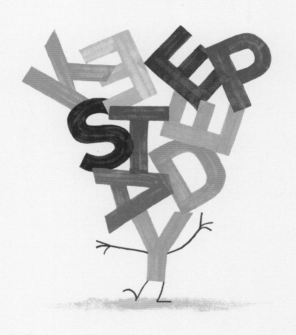

ERIK MARINOVICH

www.thebiganimals.com

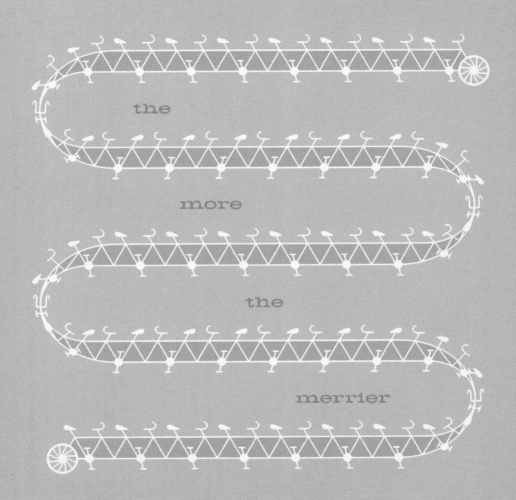

the
more
the
merrier

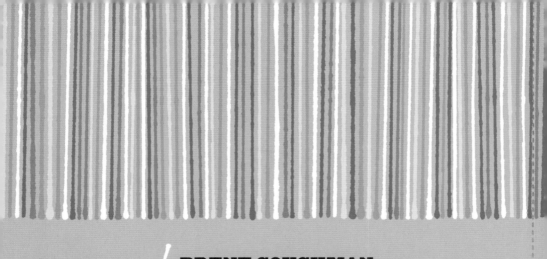

live now
www.welivenow.org

**BRENT COUCHMAN
DESIGN & ILLUSTRATION**
www.brentcouchman.com

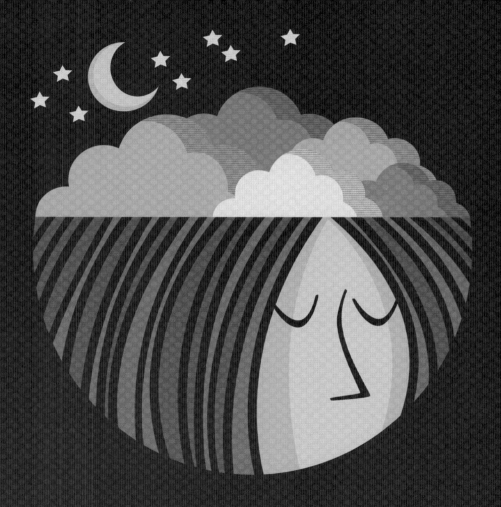

KNOWONDER

live now
www.welivenow.org

/

CHRISTOPHER DAVID RYAN
www.cdryan.com

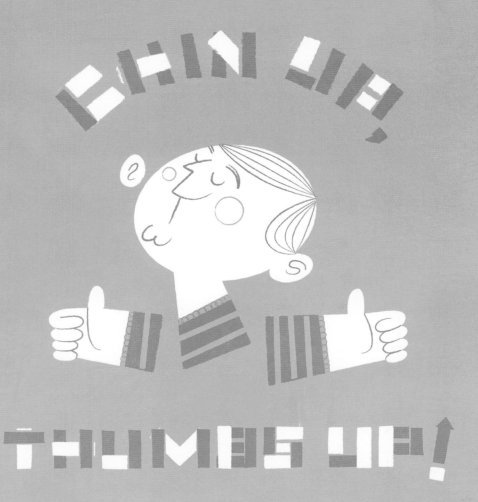

live now
www.welivenow.org

/

LYDIA NICHOLS
www.lydianichols.com

~~This Page~~
LIVE
~~Intentionally~~
~~Left Blank~~

live now
www.welivenow.org

MIKEY BURTON
www.mikeyburton.com

live now
www.welivenow.org

ERIC SMITH
www.idrawallday.com

Be CHEERFUL FRIEND

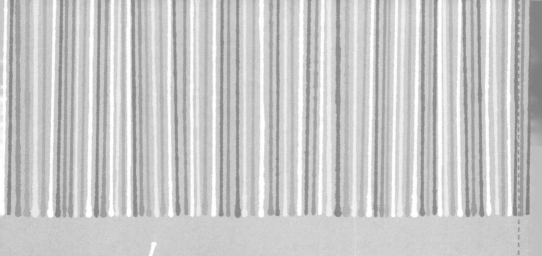

live now
www.welivenow.org

ERIC SMITH
www.idrawallday.com

STAY IN TOUCH

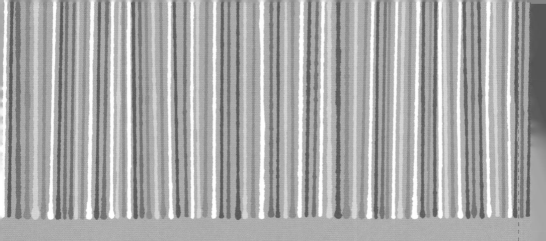

live now **/** **LUKE BOTT**

www.welivenow.org
www.lukebott.com

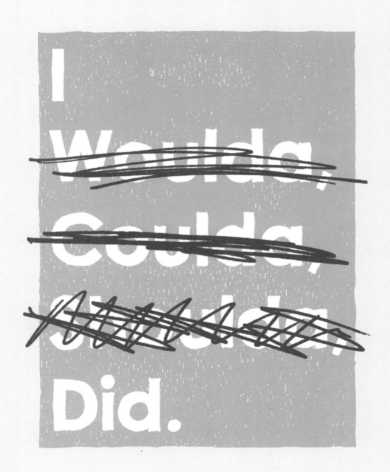

live now
www.welivenow.org

JESSE HORA
www.jessehora.com

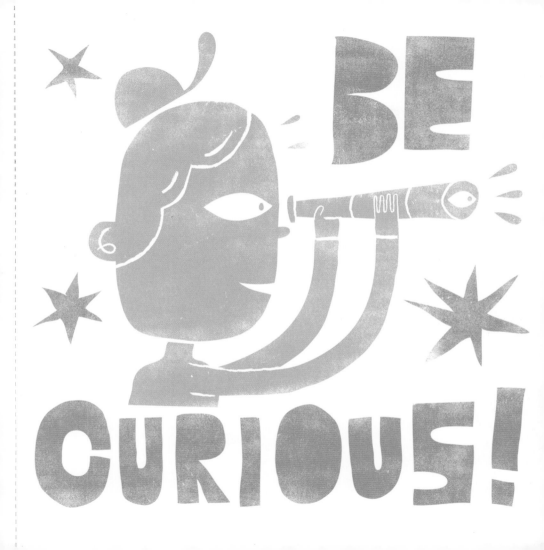

live now
www.welivenow.org

/

BEN ASLETT
www.benaslett.co.uk

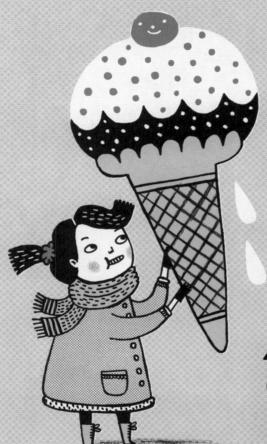

YOU deserve GOOD THINGS.

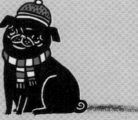

GEMMA CORRELL

www.gemmacorrell.com

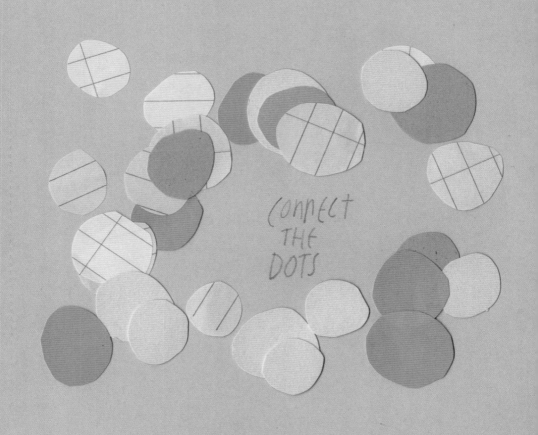

CONNECT
THE
DOTS

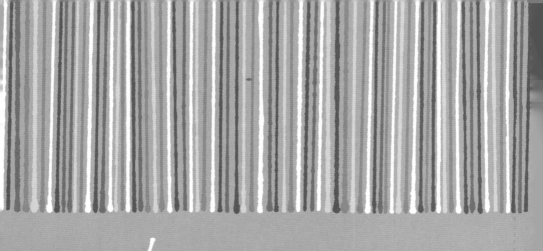

live now
www.welivenow.org

/

ERIC SMITH
www.idrawallday.com

SPECTACULARS
DELICIOUS LOVELY fresh cut grass
THE LAST COOKIE
AFTERNOON NAP
FIND
LEISURE
DELIGHT
COOL
BREEZE
IN THE LITTLE
SUPER
THINGS
GOOD
daydreaming the BEST
BOOK
DELIGHT
Jolly APPLE PIE
lemonade

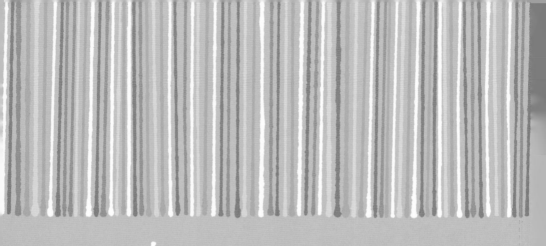

live now
www.welivenow.org

GILLIAN MACLEOD
www.gillianmacleod.com

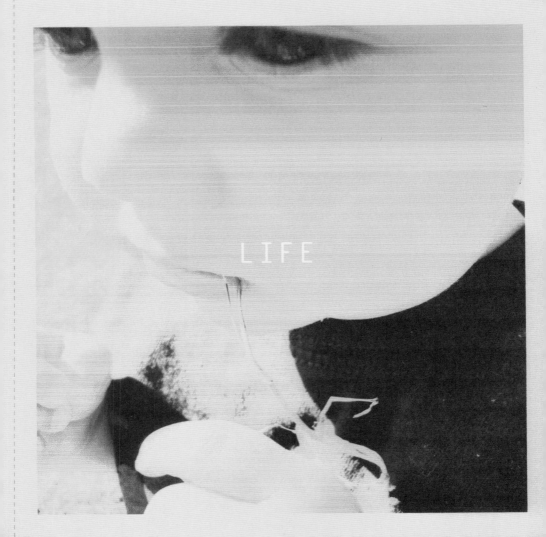

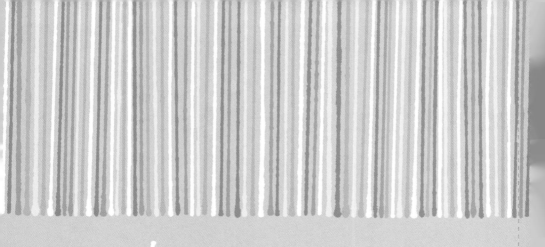

live now
www.welivenow.org

/

ERIC SMITH
www.idrawallday.com

FREE TO RESPOND WITH A SMILE

ANTON WEFLÖ

www.antonweflo.com

Treat your friends
like your family,
and your family
like your friends.

live now
www.welivenow.org

DAVID GIBSON
www.david-gibson.co.uk

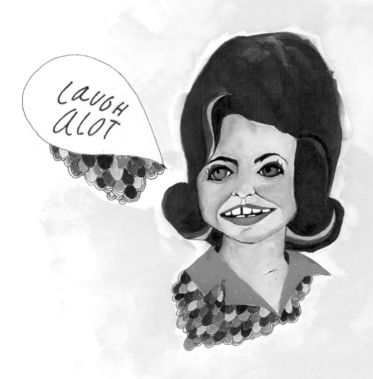

live now
www.welivenow.org

JANINE WAREHAM
janinewareham.com

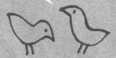

JIM DATZ
www.neitherfishnorfowl.com

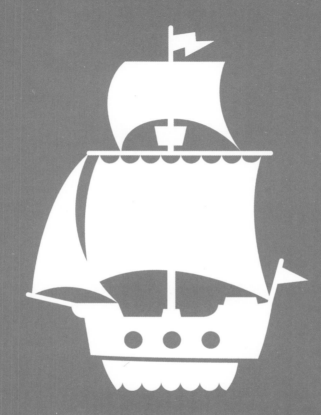

FRIEND
SHIP

live now
www.welivenow.org

/

EMIL KOZAK
www.emilkozak.com

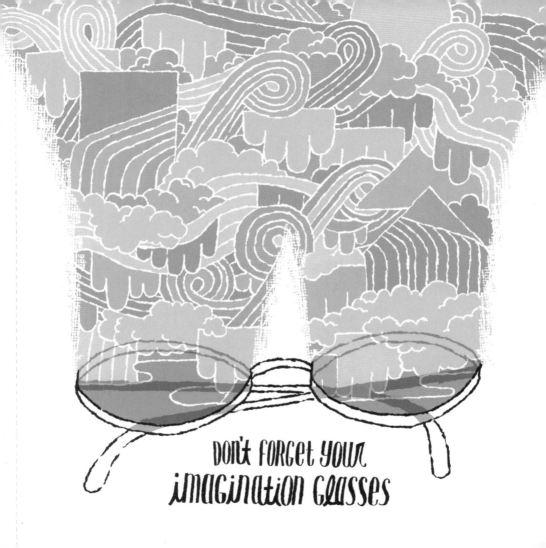

don't forget your
imagination glasses

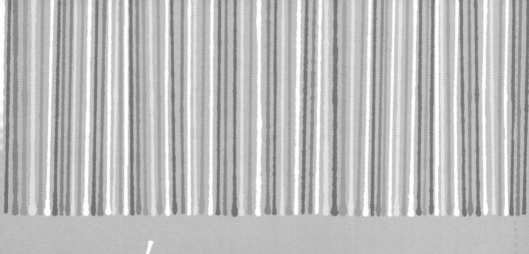

live now

www.welivenow.org

/

SLIDE SIDEWAYS

www.slide-sideways.com

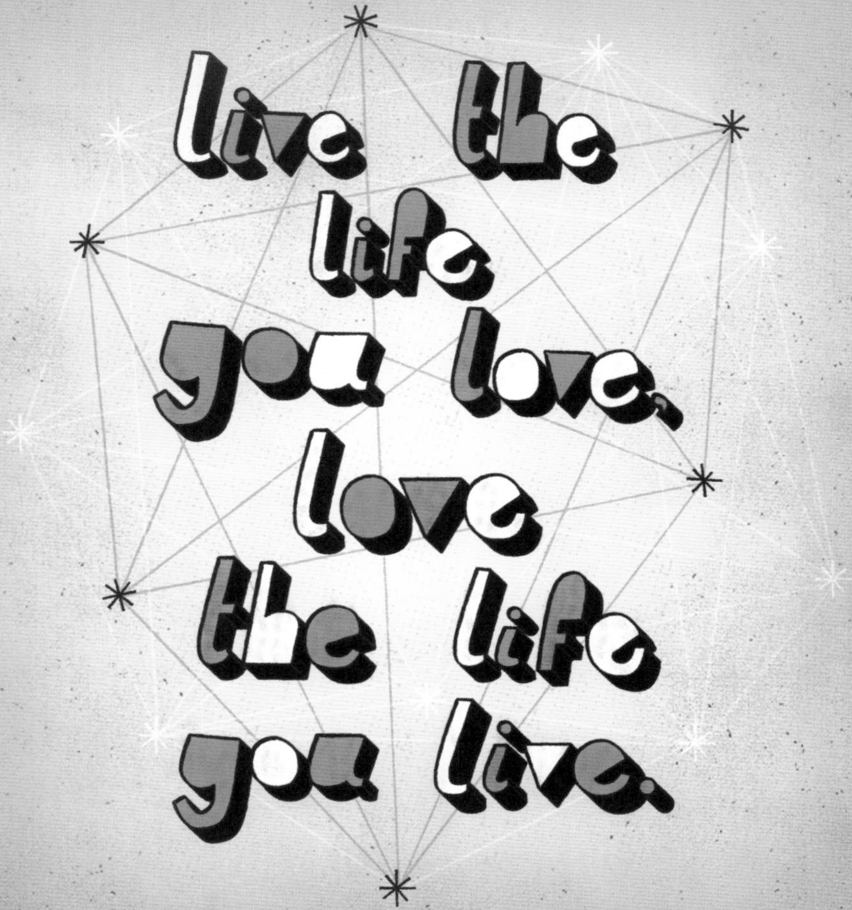
live the
life
you love,
love
the life
you live.

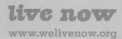
www.welivenow.org

SCOTT ALBRECHT
www.ScottyFiveAlive.com

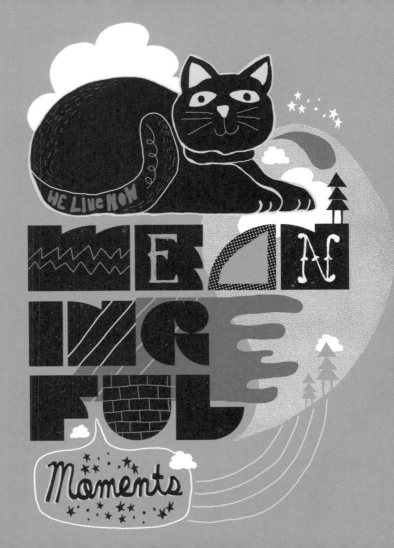

KEVIN "CONOR" KELLER

www.themischiefco.com

FULL OF BELIEF

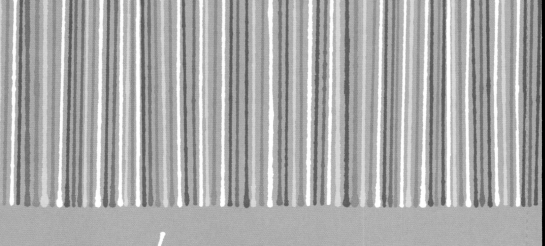

live now
www.welivenow.org

/

THE SILENT GIANTS
www.thesilentgiants.com

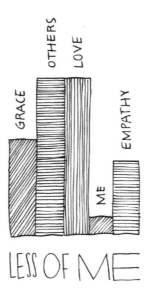

GRACE OTHERS LOVE ME EMPATHY

LESS OF ME

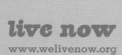
www.welivenow.org

/

CHELSEY SCHEFFE
www.chelseyscheffe.com

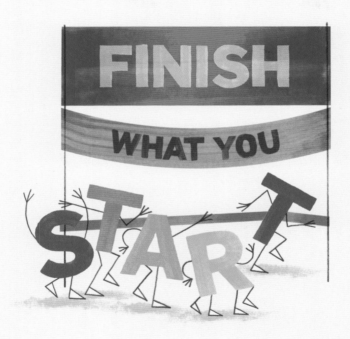

live now
www.welivenow.org

/

ERIK MARINOVICH
www.thebiganimals.com

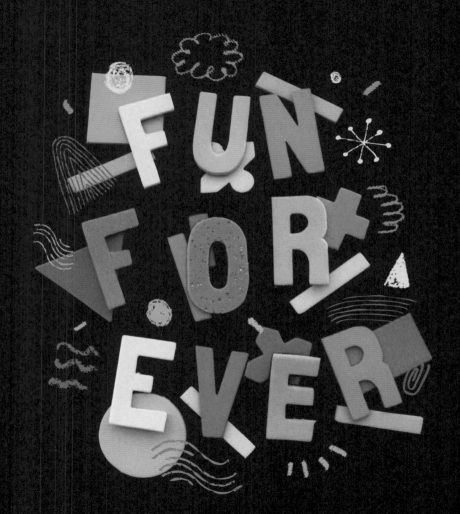

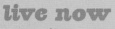

www.welivenow.org

BOSQUE STUDIO

www.holabosque.com.ar

TRUE HAPPINESS IS GIVING IT away

KATE MISS

www.katemiss.com, www.forme-foryou.com

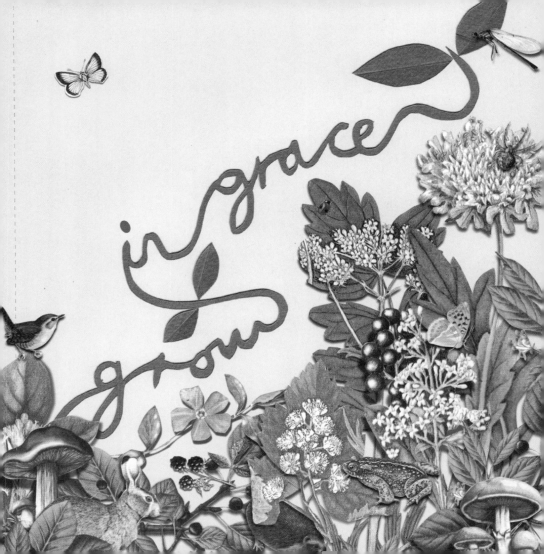

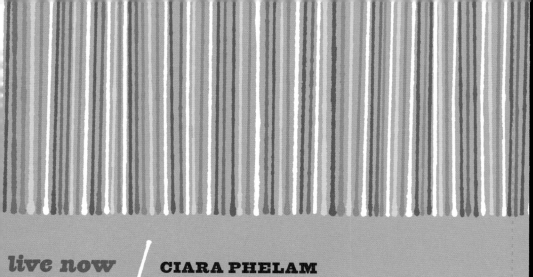

live now
www.welivenow.org

/

CIARA PHELAM
www.iamciara.co.uk

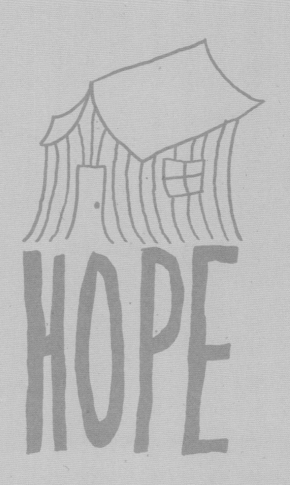

live now
www.welivenow.org

/

ERIC SMITH
www.idrawallday.com

Treat every person you meet today like they are the most important person in the world.

live now
www.welivenow.org

/

ERIC SMITH
www.idrawallday.com

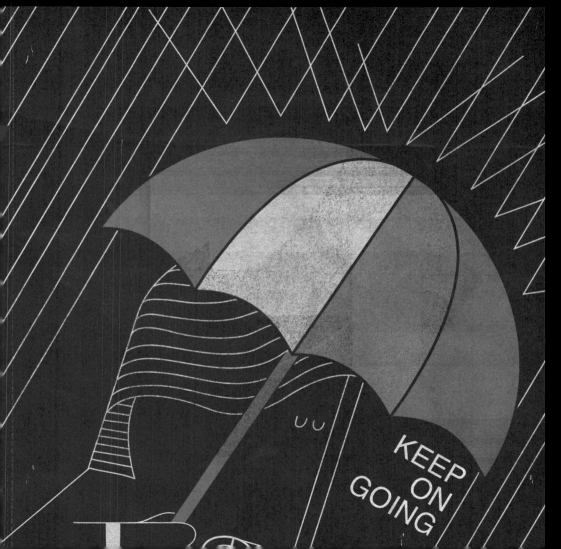

KEEP
ON
GOING

live now
www.welivenow.org

/

DALE EDWIN MURRAY
www.daleedwinmurray.com

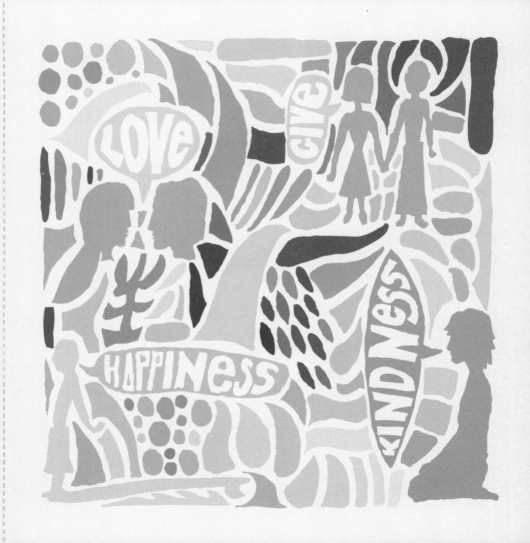

CHRIS ROBB
www.chrisrobb.com

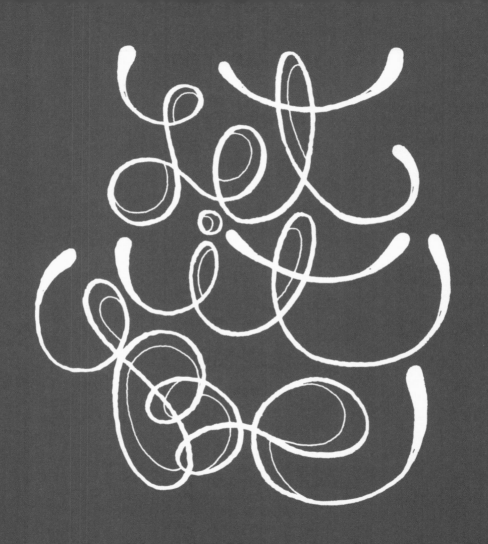

live now
www.welivenow.org

/

ASHKAHN SHAHPARNIA
www.Ashkahn.com

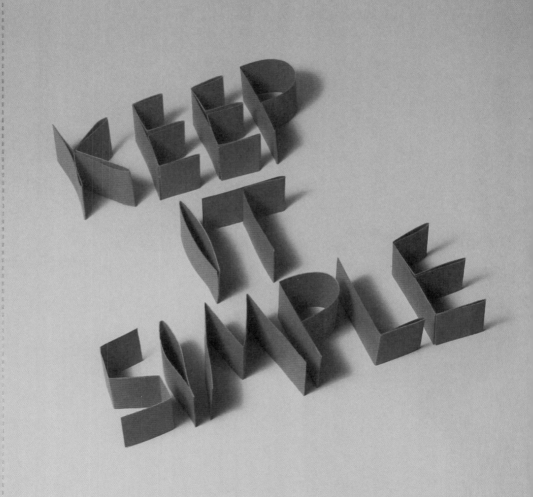

live now / **ISTVÁN VASIL**
www.welivenow.org   www.istvanvasil.com

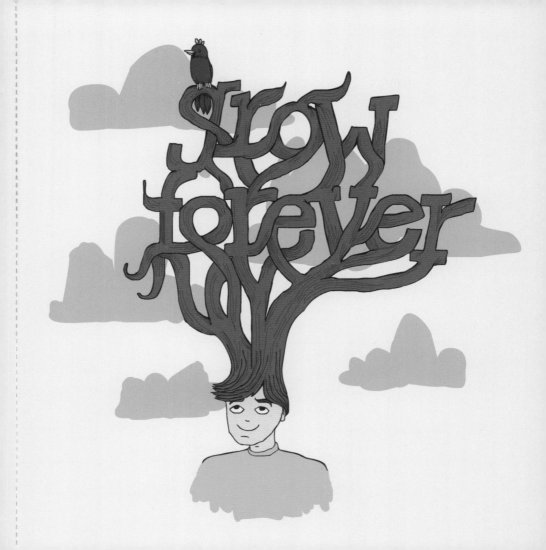

live now
www.welivenow.org

/

MIRIAMPERSAND
www.miriampersand.com, www.unabuenabarba.com

IT IS WHAT IT IS

YOU MAKE IT

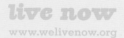
www.welivenow.org

BRENT COUCHMAN
DESIGN & ILLUSTRATION

www.brentcouchman.com

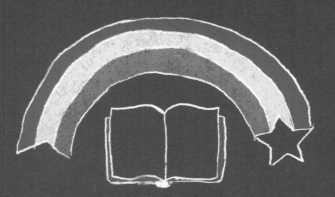

ALWAYS

LEARNING

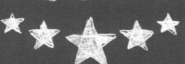

live now
www.welivenow.org

/

JOE VAN WETERING
www.joevw.com

LOVE

live now
www.welivenow.org

/

HIJIRI K. SHEPHERD
www.hijirik.com

LET'S MAKE TIME FOR ALL THE THINGS WE WANT TO DO.

live now
www.welivenow.org

/

SCOTT ALBRECHT
www.ScottyFiveAlive.com

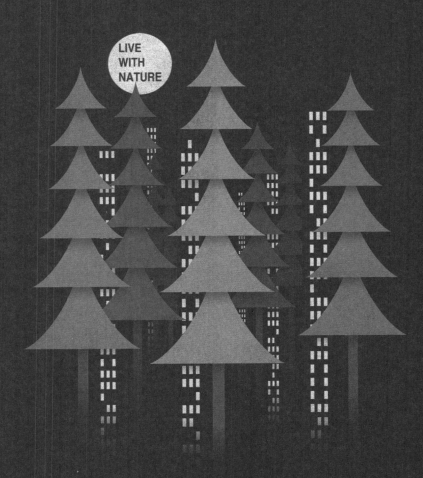

live now
www.welivenow.org

/

DALE EDWIN MURRAY

www.daleedwinmurray.com

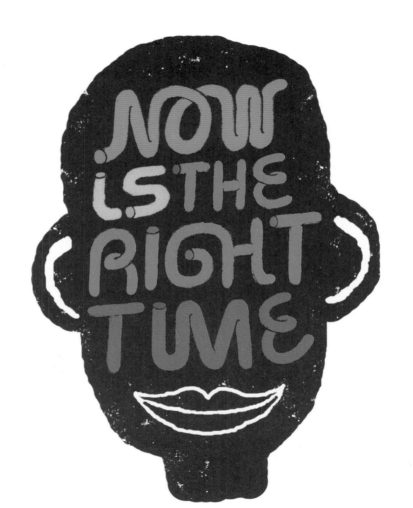

live now / **JULIAN PEÑA**

www.welivenow.org www.flickr.com/punagraphic

MAKE YOUR OWN KIND OF MUSIC

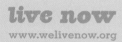
live now
www.welivenow.org

DAN CASSARO
www.YoungJerks.com

ALWAYS LOVE ALLWAYS

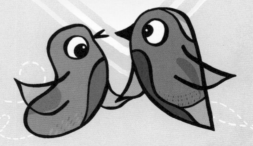

always love, all ways

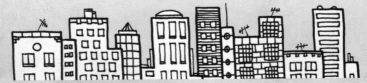

live now

CARLO PAOLO ESPIRITU
www.wildnice.com

SELL EVERYTHING AND BUY WISDOM.

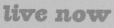

live now
www.welivenow.org

/

ERIC SMITH
www.idrawallday.com

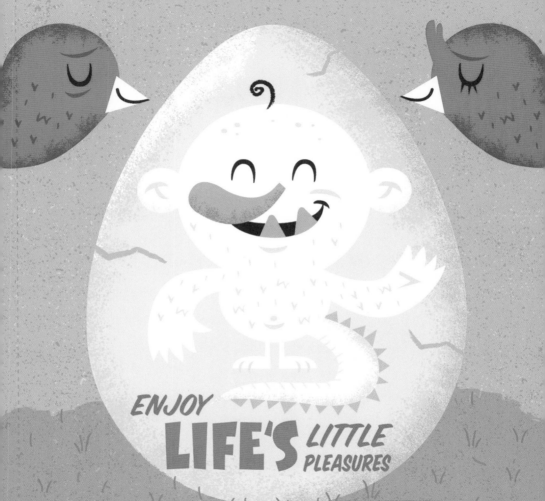

live now
www.welivenow.org

/

TAD CARPENTER
www.tadcarpenter.com

ROLL
UP YOUR
SLEEVES

live now
www.welivenow.org

/

ERIC SMITH
www.idrawallday.com

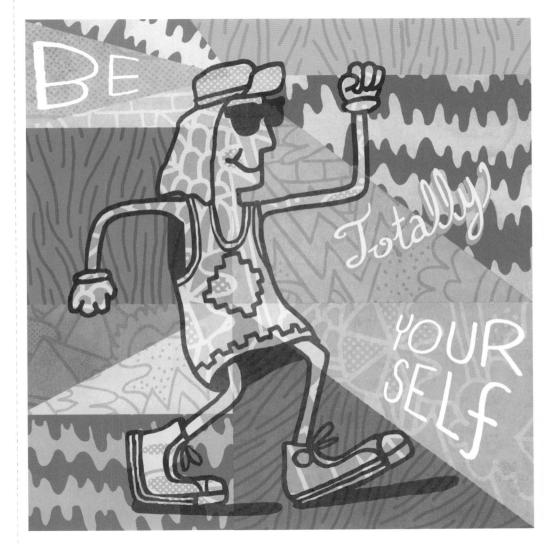

live now
www.welivenow.org

/

WILL BRYANT
www.willbryant.com

MALAYSIA 15¢

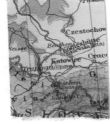

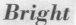

Bright

AV 627247
319 NINE

SAFETY MATCHES
JANATA
THAYAMMAL MATCH WORKS,
EATTUR—K·V·I·

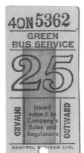

4ON 5362
GREEN
BUS SERVICE
25
INWARD   OUTWARD
Issued
subject to
Company's
Rules and
Regulations
CONTROL SYSTEMS LTD.
2180

PHILEMON

1-3 I, Paul, am a prisoner for the sake of Christ, here with my brother Timothy. I write this letter to you, Philemon, my good friend and companion in this work—also to our sister Apphia, to Archippus, a real trooper, and to the church that meets in your house. God's best to you! Christ's blessings on you!

4-7 Every time your name comes up in my prayers, I say, "Oh, thank you, God!" I keep hearing of the love and faith you have for the Master Jesus, which brings over to other Christians. And I keep praying that this faith we build in common keeps showing up in the good things we do, and that people recognize Christ in all of it. Friend, you have no idea how good your love makes me feel, doubly so when I see your hospitality to fellow believers.

To Call the Slave Your Friend

8-9 In line with all this I have a favor to ask of you. As Christ's ambassador and now a prisoner for him, I wouldn't hesitate to command this if I thought it necessary, but I'd rather make it a personal request.

10-14 While here in jail, I've fathered a child, so to speak. And here he is, hand-carrying this letter—Onesimus! He was useless to you before, now he's useful to both of us. I'm sending him back to you, but it feels like I'm cutting off my right arm in doing so. I wanted in the worst way to keep him here as your stand-in to

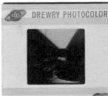

DREWRY PHOTOCOLOR

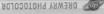

DREWRY PHOTOCOLOR

Relax

live now
www.welivenow.org

/

ANTHONY ZINONOS
www.anthonyzinonos.com

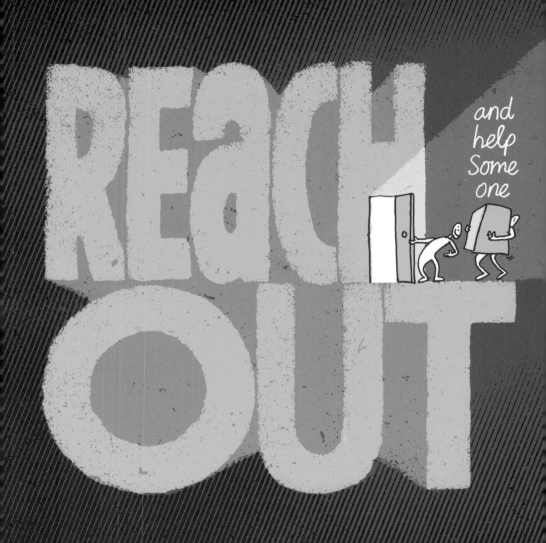

live now

/

ANDY SMITH
www.asmithillustration.com

RECYCLE

LOVE

live now

/

CELESTE PREVOST

celesteprevost.com

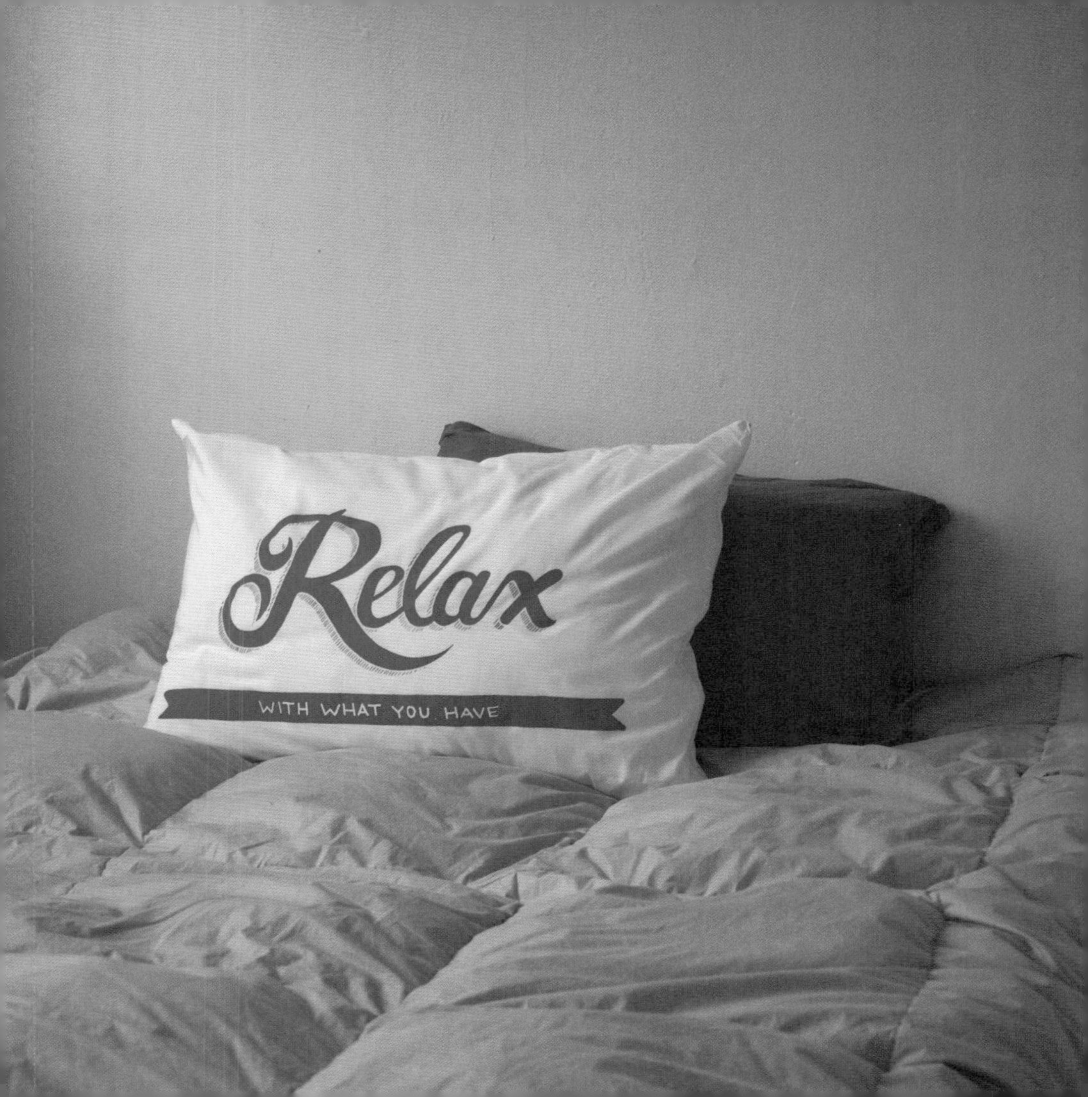
Relax
WITH WHAT YOU HAVE

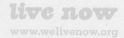
www.welivenow.org

CHAD KOURI
www.longliveanalog.com, www.thepostfamily.com

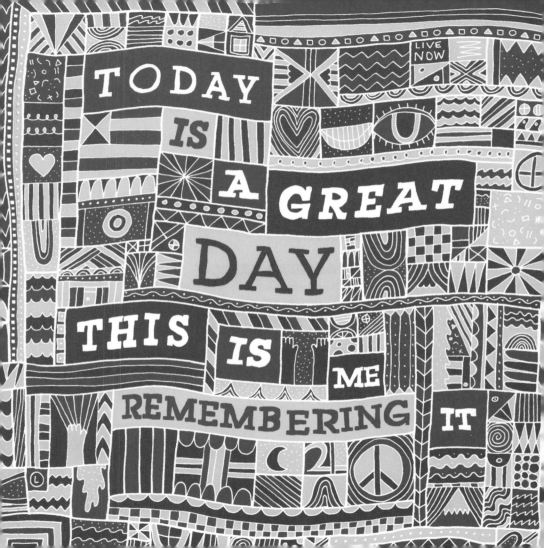

live now
www.welivenow.org

/

BIJAN BERAHIMI
www.bijanberahimi.com

I'm thankful.
for you!

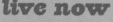

live now
www.welivenow.org

/

ERIC SMITH
www.idrawallday.com

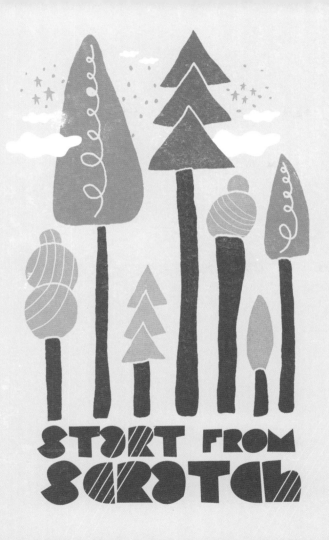

START FROM SCRATCH

KEVIN "CONOR" KELLER

www.themischiefco.com

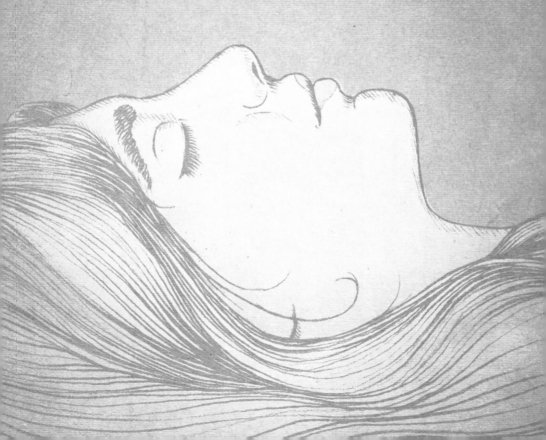

CLOSE YOUR EYES
AND FEEL THE SUN
SHIMMER.

live now
www.welivenow.org

KELLY SHEROD
www.kellysteven.com

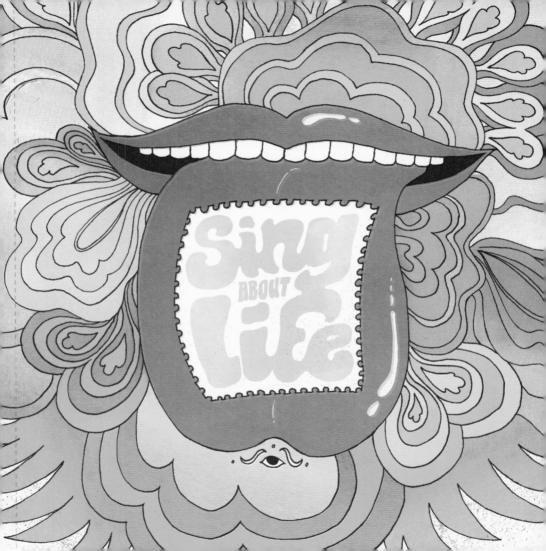

live now
www.welivenow.org

/

ERIK ANTHONY HAMLINE

www.woodsandweather.com, www.steadyprintshop.com

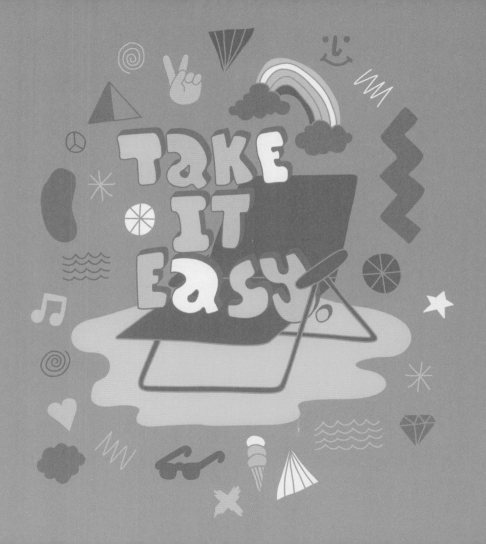

live now
www.welivenow.org

/

COREY THOMPSON
www.thisiscoreythompson.com

COMMON UNITY

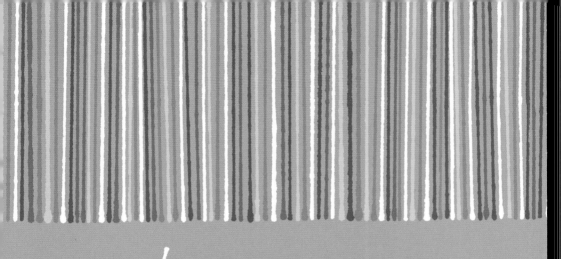

live now
www.welivenow.org

/

CHRIS CLARKE
www.chris-clarke.co.uk

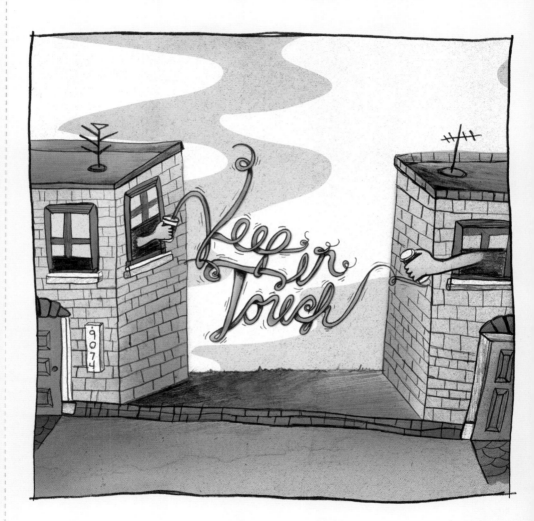

RYAN DOGGENDORF

doganddwarf.com

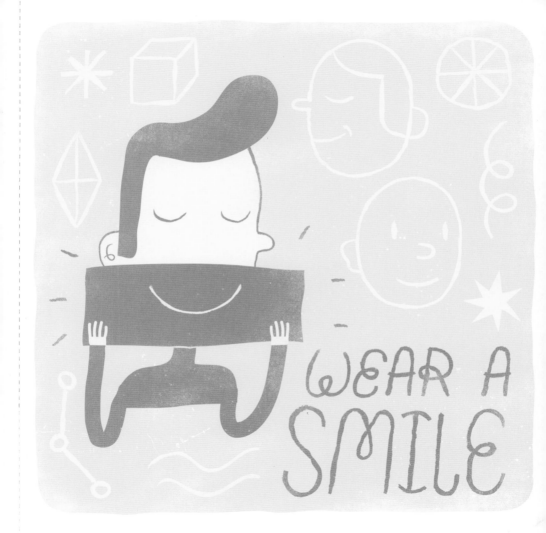

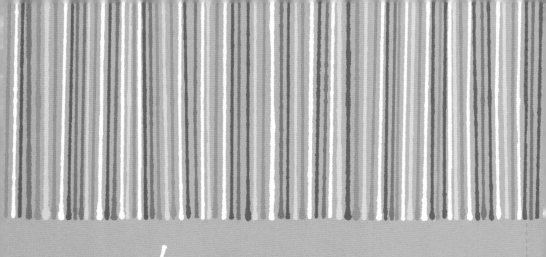

live now
www.welivenow.org

/

BEN ASLETT
www.benαslett.co.uk